Legal & Disclaimer

The information contained in this book is not designed to replace or take the place of any form of medication or professional medical advice. The information in this book has been provided for educational and entertainment purposes only.

The information contained in this book has been compiled from sources deemed reliable, and it is accurate to the best of the Author's knowledge. However, the Author cannot guarantee its accuracy and validity so cannot be held liable for any errors or omissions. Changes are periodically made to this book. You must consult your doctor or get professional medical advice before using any of the suggested remedies, techniques, or information in this book.

Upon using the information contained in this book, you agree to hold harmless the Author from and against any damages, costs and expenses, including any legal fees, potentially resulting from the application of any of the information provided by this guide. This disclaimer applies to any damages or injury caused by the use and application, whether directly or indirectly, of any advice or information presented, whether for breach of contract, tort, negligence, personal injury, criminal intent, or under any other cause of action.

You agree to accept all the risks of using the information presented inside this book. You need to consult a professional medical practitioner in order to ensure you are both able & healthy enough to participate in this program.

Contents

Introduction

Essential Oils are wonderful multi-purpose beautiful smelling main ingredient in Aromatherapy – the art of using essential oils for healing and health. Allergies, a real nuisance, are a reaction from your body when an outside substance enters your body that your body does not want there. Most of us associate allergies with running noses, sour throats, sore and watery eyes; as well as other symptoms like fatigue. Essential oils can be used in your daily life throughout the whole year to help alleviate allergy symptoms as well as in some cases eliminate them.

There are various kinds of essential oils, and there is a bit of confusion as to what an essential oil is and the carrier oils that you mix to use with the essentials properly. This guide will help you understand all about the oils; how to use and prepare them. The brand of essential oil is very important because not all essential oils are the same. You have to be very careful when purchasing your oils because if they are not correctly made, then you will not get all the wonderful benefits of the essential oil experience.

On the brighter side, you are entering a world of creating a wonderfully scented house, so that when people walk in through your door they are going to inhale a beautiful scent and want to know what it is. People will remember you because when they walked into your house they felt good. Another benefit of essential oils is not only making yourself feel good, but you will make others feel good as well, which will daily change our mood and stress level. A good mood and lower stress level will help you feel happy and healthy.

Though essential oils cannot help you with everything, but where this oil cannot help, it is strongly advised you see a doctor. Natural medicine is excellent for preventive measures and reducing ailments that already exist if proper instruction and long term commitments are followed. Though it is strongly suggested that if you suspect any allergy that is more than what an essential oil can help, then you need to see your doctor for help. Natural medicine is wonderful, but sometimes conventional medicine is needed in the event that something in the body had gotten out of hand. The thing that natural medicine cannot always help is illnesses brought on by genetic problems. Some problems are just too strong to heal through normal practices. This is perfectly fine. The whole point is you getting better, healed, and balanced for peace of mind.

Essential oils are a part of holistic healing. Wellness and taking care of the whole body is an ancient healing practice, and it still works today. Your well-being is of the utmost importance for longevity. Being allergy free as well helps you look and feel youthful and live comfortably well. Essential oils can help you cure allergies by following some pretty simple routines and recipes. You will have the benefit of being healed as well as smelling really good. Who doesn't like a good smelling person? You will not only feel good that you are allergy free, but your mood and facial

expressions change when your sense of smell is tantalizing with something you like. Between lemon, lavender, clove, and many more essential oils, there is bound to be a few essential oils that you will love.

Now let us take a look at the beautiful essence of essential oils, and all the wonderful aromas you have to choose from. Through this guide, you will better understand what makes a good essential oil as well as all the wonderful places you can use essential oils. Places like in your home, your car, at your office, as beauty products, and more. Hopefully, the insight you will learn here will guide you to a new lifestyle that will incorporate essential oils throughout your day so you can aim for an allergy free life.

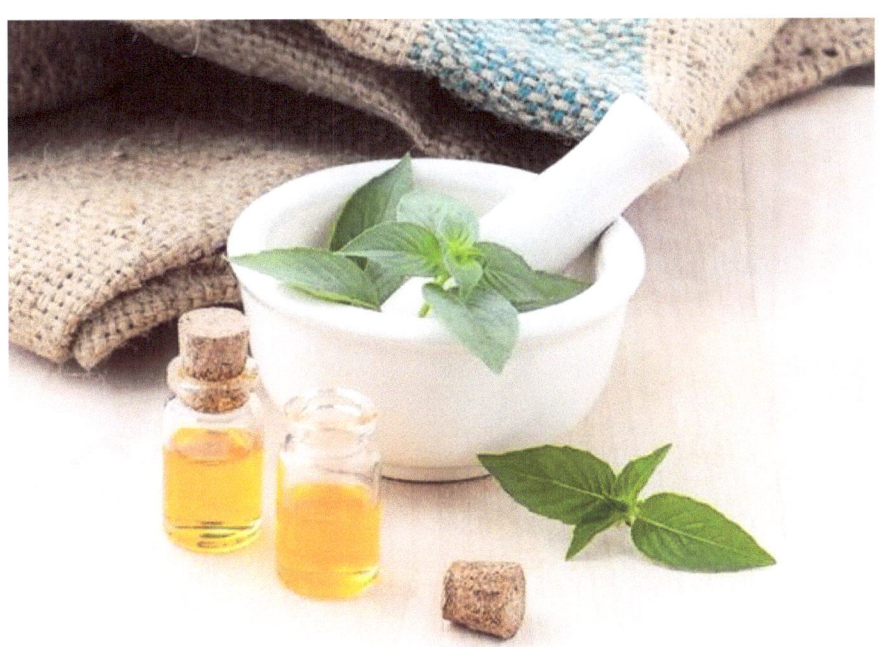

Special Bonus

To thank you for purchasing my guide, I have specifically prepared the bonus **"Aromatherapy – First Aid Kit"** report for you. This report will show you how you can heal yourself inside out using the power of aromatherapy.

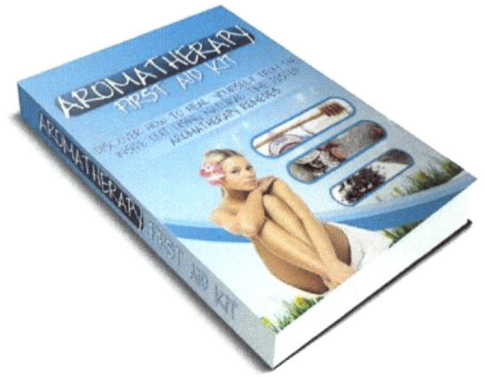

Inside this report, you will find:

1. Secrets to a natural beauty and great looking skin

2. How you can make your own perfumes and hair care treatment

3. And many more….

To download this special bonus, simply visit this URL below:

http://giveaway.kindleheaven.com/index.php/essential-oils-aromatherapy/

….And put in both your name and email there so I know who to address and which email address to send the report to

Chapter 1: What Are Allergies?

Allergies are the human response to allergens that exist around us all the time. Pollen in the trees, dander from our pets, specific allergens in our foods, drinks, and medications.

You can find allergens in your environment and also in your foods, drinks, and medications. Allergens can shake up a person's immune system and cause some symptoms in the body. Signs of being irritated by allergens can take years to show up, but when symptoms of allergies show up they can be from mild to severe, but you know something not right when they are there.

You will notice things like coughing, itchiness in your nose or eyes, swollen and watery eyes as well as other eye problems. Food allergies can happen in many different forms. The scary thing with food allergies is that you ingest something, and you have so many different areas of your internal system that can be sensitive.

Swelling is one sign of food allergies. Swelling of your throat, lips, face, or tongue. You can easily vomit if you are allergic to some foods. Skin reactions such as peeling skin, itchy skin, and rashes can also be allergic reactions you might experience.

The truth about allergies is that it is not the allergen that causes the bad reaction, it is actually a person's immune system that is harmful to them, because the immune system overreacts to most harmless allergens. Things like histamine and antibodies are used to get rid of what the body recognizes as a very harmful substance that really may just be simple pollen.

The importance of keeping your immune system working in top form is the utmost importance to keeping your body from overacting to allergens. You see people who go through life with not a care in the world when the pollen season is around. Please remember one very specific thing and that is moderation is the key to all balance and health. So if you are outside for too long and not getting enough rest, you just may start to suffer from allergies. There are things in life you may want to do but if you do not properly protect yourself, your body will punish you.

Essential oils help with your immune system in more ways than one. But before we discover all the amazing ways essential oils can help with allergies, it is very important to point out that you have a responsibility to take care of your health in order to fight allergies with your immune system. No essential oil in the world is going to help you - possibly temporarily. But if you drink alcohol all day, eat greasy foods, sleep very little, and never exercise then you are setting yourself up for possibly really bad allergies.

It is essential to adopt a pretty simple, well-rounded diet of vegetable, grains, fruit, and lean proteins along with food based vitamins. You want to find an activity you love to do for about twenty minutes a day, sleep at least seven hours a night - but try eight - and have good personal relationships. When you do all these things, you give yourself the first major line of defenses to protecting your immune system. This does not mean you can't have and occasional donut and anything that may not seem so healthy, it just means that the majority of your weekly life is geared towards protecting that immune system.

Once your health is kept strong by diet, exercise, and lifestyle, then on top of that you will make your life even more protected and well with essential oils. Not only will essential oils help the immune system by lowering stress, but essential oils also have many other layers that will protect you and guide you through allergy seasons with more ease.

Allergies are irritating for anyone who suffers them, so if this book tells you a way to cure allergies it might be something worth looking into. Essential oils have been around for years and have been healing people for hundreds of years. Today is no different; essential oils can help you cure your allergies. I have to let you know though you have to put in a little extra effort. The effort is well worth it.

Why would you want to walk around with a stuffy congested chest and nose if you did not have to. Essential oils with the strong vapor activity of such plants as eucalyptus help open up the pathways of your respiratory system. Essential oils hold the key to helping live long and be allergy free.

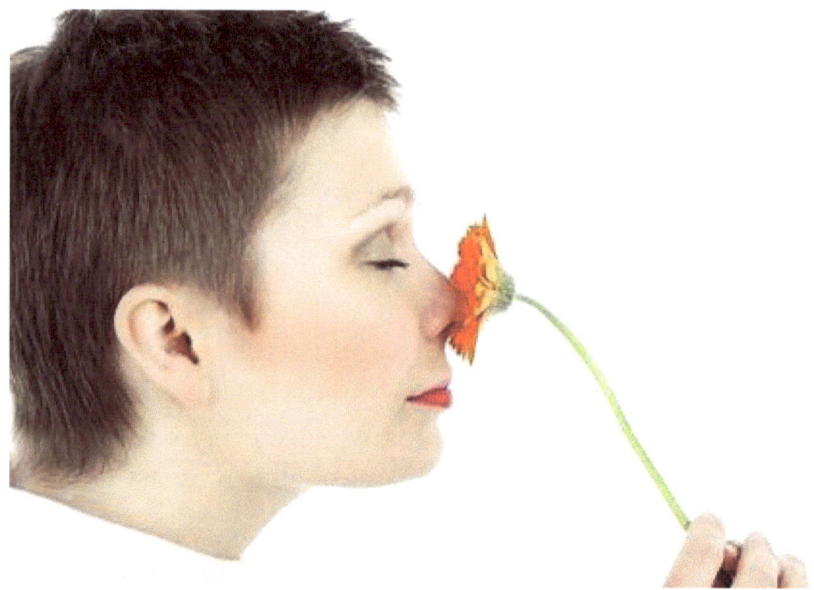

Chapter 2: Basics of Essential Oils

You might wonder where essential oils come from. Essential oils come from plants, fruits, and flowers. They are created by four different processes to take out the essence of the plant, fruit, or flower in a highly concentrated form that gets thinned out with carrier oil. When you smell the small bottle of essential oil, it is very strong because it is a very thick and heavy amount of the essential oil fragrance.

Resin tapping, cold pressing, oil extraction, and steam distillation are all ways the companies use to be able to get the essential oil from the plants, fruits, and flowers and put it into a small bottle you can buy at the natural food store or online. The one that most companies use is steam distillation. Basically, these methods take the real plant and take the very essence of the use of essential oils.

It is important for healing and health that you purchase good quality essential oils that are extracted from the healthiest plants, fruits, and flowers. There are approved companies you can be confident that they have used the purist plants to make their essential oils. This guide will give you some respected brands that have been in business for years later on in the chapters.

When you buy a little bottle of good quality essential oil, you may think it is a bit high priced, but the reality is that essential oils are so concentrated that you only need a very small amount to create the scent that you want.

You will also be mixing the essential oil with something else to thin it out. The little bottle will go a long way. Carrier oils as they call them are what you will be mixing the essential oil with. Carrier oils include grape seed oil, olive oil, coconut oil, jojoba oils and more.

There are many ways that essential oils can be used even beyond helping allergies. One excellent way is topically on your skin. Whatever you put on your skin absorbs into your body and ends up in your bloodstream. Essential oils and carrier oils are excellent to put on your skin because they are plant based, and you gain many benefits by rubbing them into your skin.

So you're rubbing something natural into your skin that your body will love. Then it absorbs the natural nutrients into your system and helps heal and maintain health along with your other health practices. On top of that, you will smell good as well.

You can also you use essential oils on your skin, hair, and body, as well as in your home, car, and if allowed your office, and you will be doing yourself some good. The good you are doing is keeping yourself away from the harmful chemicals that can easily dominate your life if you choose to let them. If you have noticed and looked at room sprays and cleaning products that are not of the natural industry, you see the chemicals that dominate the ingredient list. The fewer products you have around you that consists of the chemicals, it is a very important step in keeping yourself away from the adverse effect of allergens.

Now you are a little more familiar with what an essential oil is. It is a concentrated reduced form of wonderful healthy plants, herbs, fruit, and flowers that either have a strong or mild scent with healing properties that can be used on your body or in your home among other places.

The use of essential oils helps promote health by using them in replacement for products that otherwise have harmful chemicals that can lower your immune system opening you up to the unhealthy reaction of your body to allergens. Let's take a closer look at these chemicals that essential oil will help you stay away from.

When you go to the natural food store to buy your essential oils, you will find a few choices. You can rest assured that if they are in the natural food store and have the proper labeling from a reputable company that has been around for years, these are probably going to be very effective essential oils.

If you are looking to save a bit of money, you can choose the scents that you like and the brands that you like and then look at the different options online that can save you money. It is worth it; though you may feel like you are spending a lot at first, but you do save in the long run, and you feel so much better.

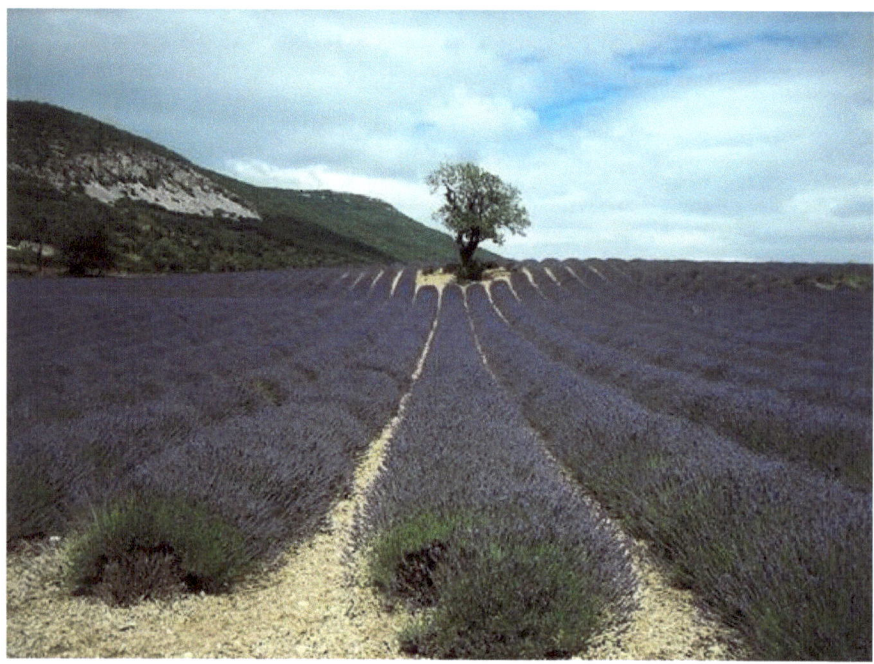

Chapter 3: Allergy Irritants from Chemical and Nature

The stores are full of products with chemicals in the food that we eat, the bathroom products we use, the make-up, the cleaning products for our homes, our clothes, and elsewhere. Big money corporations have been in business for years, advertising and putting up bright colors on things, pulling the wool over our eyes by charging us for chemicals that make us sick.

The chemicals are in small doses so they can be approved, but when the years go by and the buildup of the tiny residue that our bodies can't break down build up, we have a problem with no one to blame, and the corporations have run off with all our money.

Allergies can so easily be kicked up by these chemicals. Have you ever seen people complaining of itchy skin when they put on a shirt with a strong detergent? They might not think anything of the itch but the body is suffering. The person might do something else to compensate because they are uncomfortable, but not understating why. The chemical dryer sheets as well have chemicals in them. They may never really do any harm to some people, but if you are a sensitive person, then you need to stay away from those chemicals.

The home is a very easy place to inhale chemicals. Cleaning supplies, if not natural ingredients will put off chemicals that can go right into your respiratory track. Clorox bleach although very effective is very damaging to your cells. Yes, in small doses it may be okay for some persons, but for all those other people and no one knows for sure who it harms and who it doesn't.

But why take the risk when you don't have to. Also, air fresheners are of high chemicals, unless they are of the natural kind. You have to be very careful too because companies will say it is natural. They can say this yet the product may still be a chemical because they have just worked around the law with fancy wording to be able to make people buy their product.

Food that is full of chemicals is the biggest danger because we are putting the chemicals directly in our body. When you read the back of a food package, there is a long list of words that most people don't recognize. When you go to buy an organic apple from the store, you are getting an apple and no long list of chemicals.

Conventional apples or none organic may have a pesticide of GMO (genetically modified food). All these chemicals will somehow effect your body, and you can be allergic whether mildly or severely from any one of these chemicals. Medicine allergies as well can occur.

Nature itself can also be an allergy accelerator – pollen in the air from trees and flowers; pet dander can cause allergies; dust in the house, mites, and other household molds can also trigger and cause allergies. There are sources for allergies all around. It is why the first defense is to keep your immune system strong with a great diet and exercise daily.

Essential oils can help in many ways because you can replace almost all of the products that you use that have chemicals in them with essential oils, and essential oil recipes. Can you imagine if you were not breathing in or eating any chemicals? Note that not all essential oils are for eating, so during the safety chapter I will point out what essential oils are safe to eat and which are not. It may feel a little odd at first when you go shopping because you don't need to buy as much essential oils for your body and home. You will also end up saving money in some cases as well.

Here are some examples of chemicals you want to stay away from to keep allergy free. Formaldehyde resin is an example of a chemical that can aggravate allergies. Sulfur dioxide is not healthy and can cause allergic reactions. Cigarette smoke that has nicotine is terrible and can cause many respiratory problems and other severe problems in the body. Nitrogen Dioxide is no good either and can cause really bad bronchial problems. If you walk into a new building or a new anything, if it is not a green friendly place, it is almost certain there are going to be chemicals in the air that can make allergies flare up.

If you find yourself in a building where there are high chemical smells, simply carry a pack of tissue in your wallet and your favorite essential oil and put one drop on the clean and inhale while you are walking in the room or building that has the harsh chemicals. This way you are bypassing the harsh chemicals and getting very little of them in your respiratory track.

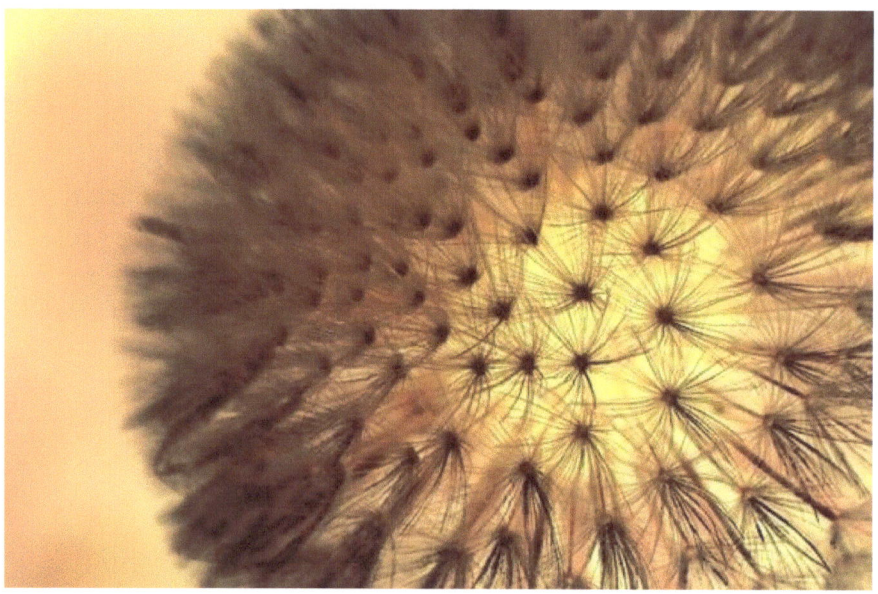

Chapter 4: Managing Allergies with Essential Oils

Essential oils can help you maintain and in some instances eliminate allergies. Do you wonder how? There are a few answers to this question, and one is quite obvious, you have to stay away from the chemicals, so when you stay away from chemicals and use essential oils in their place, you have just eliminated half the problem. It is not that difficult; you just have to train yourself to do something that you are not quite used to, but you can handle it. Why suffer when you do not have to.

Stop buying cleaning products with chemicals; that is the quickest way to stay away from chemicals. You can do two things to make sure you have every product you need that you use to buy. You can buy natural cleaning products and mix your cleaning products with essential oils. Some products are made with the essential oils, so if you do not want to take the time to mix them, you can go to the largest health food store near you, and buy their already made cleaning products with essential oils. Check out chapter seven in this guide for great recipes of essential oil cleaning products.

Using essential oils in your foods to flavor them instead of buying processed food with artificial flavors is another great way to help stay away from allergies, stop them from forming, and possibly eliminate them if you have them. Essential oils like Peppermint, grapefruit, and lavender are all essential oils you can eat, but you want to make sure that the company you buy from is giving you an essential oil that is safe to eat. The best thing to do is ask, and if they are not sure, then don't do it, but find a company that is. When in doubt simply use lemon, grapefruit, peppermint and lavender for eating from the regular grocery store or produce aisle of your natural food store.

Only buy one that is labeled safe for ingestion or just buy the real thing. Carrier oils like coconut oil and olive oil can be eaten if they are the edible kind, but if you buy from an essential oil section, make sure these are oils you can ingest.

The next way to stay away from allergies is using essential oils for skin care regimen. What you wash your face, body, hands, and hair with are all chances to be near chemicals that may cause you allergies. When you use essential oils and products that are natural and contain essential oils, you are caring for yourself by keeping yourself away from harsh chemicals. You keep them from not absorbing through your skin from chemical lotions, makeup, and cleansers, as well as through your scalp from chemical shampoos, and through your skin from make-ups or cleansers.

Almost every aspect of your life you can control how much you are exposed to harsh chemicals. By using the essential oils and the natural products that go along with them to help take care of yourself and your home, you are breathing fresh air and keeping harmful substances from inhibiting your immune system from working properly.

This is one of the ways to cure your allergies and promote a long-lasting life for yourself. There are more ways to come, but eliminating your exposure to chemicals whether inside or outside of your body and replacing what normally had chemicals with essential oils, you have probably saved yourself several trips to the doctor.

Allergies can easily depress you as well, so steering clear of unwanted chemicals and harsh preservatives can help cure your allergies and keep depression away especially in the winter months.

When it is cold outside, it is the perfect time to be indoors and cleaning with your essential oil cleaning products, as well as taking care of your body with the essential oil recipes found later on in this book.

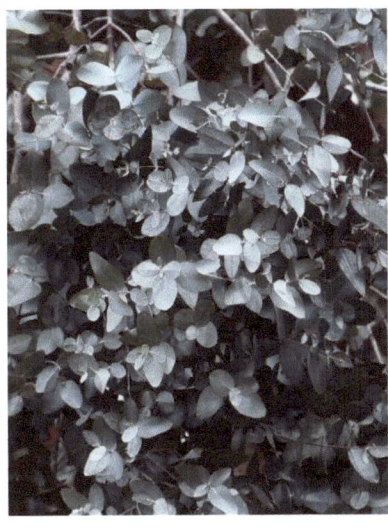

Chapter 5: Safety with Essential Oils

Safety is essential with essential oils. You are still dealing with oils and highly concentrate versions of what the label reads. You don't want to put essential oils in your eyes. You want to be cautious to of what type of essential oils you are buying. As stated earlier, there are only a few essential oils you can ingest, but not all essential oils that you are allowed to be ingested can be ingested. Like you may be able to pick up lavender essential oil you can eat, but then they also make lavender ones you can't ingest. The bottle must say that you can eat the oil.

Good essential oils run from six dollars up to thirty dollars. They do make dollar store version essential oils, but you do not want to use these because they are not the safest. They are not extracted from the plants. They are cheap chemical versions that can harm you. Never try to drink or ingest an essential oil from a dollar store.

Aura Cacia is one of the most trusted names in essential oils. All the major natural food stores carry this brand. The scent and purity of their products are wonderful. When you open their bottle, you will be so pleased with the result. They make beautiful products and use all the highest quality ways of extracting and growing. This is a safe brand to use.

Essential oils, just because they are natural do not mean that there is not a way for them to be harmful. As a rule, you do not want to ingest an essential oil, of course there are exceptions, but if you are unclear just say no. As with nature, you may have reactions to particular essential oils.

You have to stop using an essential oil if your skin swells, or you have any bad reaction to an essential oil. You buy them in a highly concentrate form, so you use just one to a few small drop in a diluting solution depending on what you are doing.

You always want to be cautious and aware when using any product. Essential oils are no different. Just be careful when you are mixing them as well, wash your hands after using them. You do not want to rub oil in your eyes. When used with caution and understanding, essential oils are great ways to keep your home allergen-free so that you can live freely.

Another safety precaution with the essential oils is that of staining. You want to be careful when you spray your room, as well as when you put the oil on your body. You don't want to stain your clothes or your furniture and fabric in your home. So if you need to find a space that is not noticeable, spray your spray there.

The best case scenario is to put the essential oils on before you go to sleep, so the oil as ample time to soak in. You can also protect your neck with a towel, as well as only rub the essential oil into your body long before you put your clothes on. It is just a precaution. Oils do absorb into the skin if you need just to take any excess off.

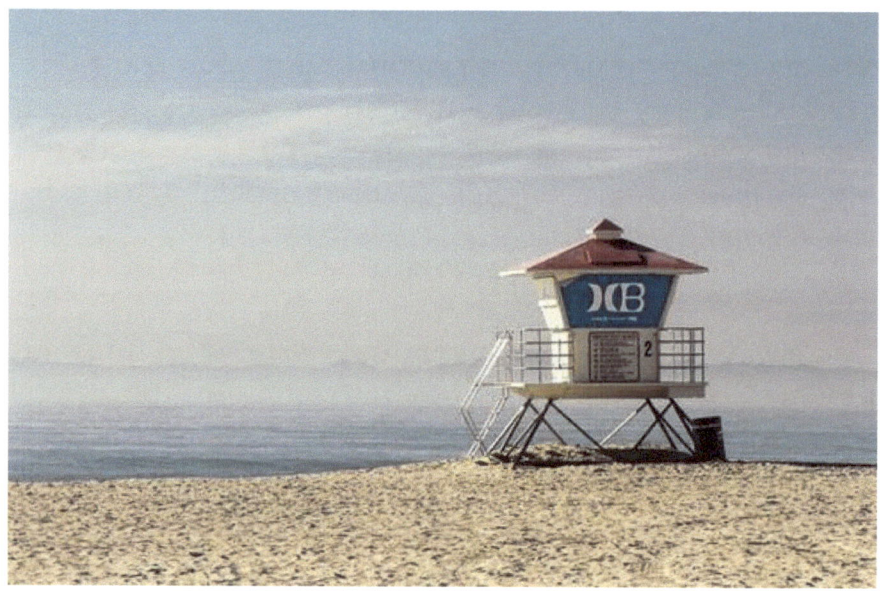

Chapter 6: Curing Allergies with Essential Oils

Curing your allergies with essential oils is quite simple. You simply follow the steps for using essential oils throughout your entire life. With home, beauty regimens, as well as eating a diet rich in vegetables, fruits, and grains. Also incorporate lean proteins as well. The next chapter is going to give you recipes that will help cure your allergies that usually affect your respiratory and skin.

Eucalyptus

Eucalyptus is one of the most effective essential oils for curing your allergies. When you use eucalyptus for opening up your breathing passages, it helps during the strongest allergy seasons, which are fall and spring when the pollen from the trees are blowing in the air. Eucalyptus is an anti-inflammatory and helps with respiratory conditions and headaches. You need only to mix it with grape seed oil and rub the combination on your chest and throat. You will smell really nice and natural. You will also feel great because of the clarity from which you can breathe.

Lemon

Lemon is another excellent respiratory essential oil that will help cure allergies. Since most allergies happen in the lung, throat, mouth, and nose area, all these essential oils that cure allergies are for the respiratory track. Lemon cleanses everything and everywhere. Lemon can be used both topically and if you buy a lemon essential oil that is approved for eating you can take it for the allergies internally as well. It is antibacterial and it reduces inflammation associated with the respiratory track.

Ginger

Ginger is a good essential oil for curing allergies. It is more for digestion, but it is still very effective for healing the respiratory track. Coughing can be eliminated, and breathing can become clearer and good with ginger essential oil. Ginger in the food form from the produce aisle plus essential oil ginger rubbed on topically with the carrier oil is very effective.

Peppermint

Peppermint essential oil helps cure allergies. It is strong and wonderful for allowing the sinuses to open up and be clear from allergies. You can put the peppermint on a towel with a carrier oil and wrap that towel around the back of your neck while you work on the computer.

Lavender

Lavender is an amazing essential oil as well. The number one thing that lavender does that is important for curing allergies is that it is a natural antihistamine. Histamine, as you remember, is what your puts out to attack the area where the foreign substance is bothering you. Lavender keeps swelling down as well as working as an excellent anti-inflammatory. Lavender is very effective for the immune system as well.

This is a list of essential oils that help cure allergies. Now let us take a look at some wonderful recipes that you can follow to help cure your allergies and allergy symptoms safely and prescription free.

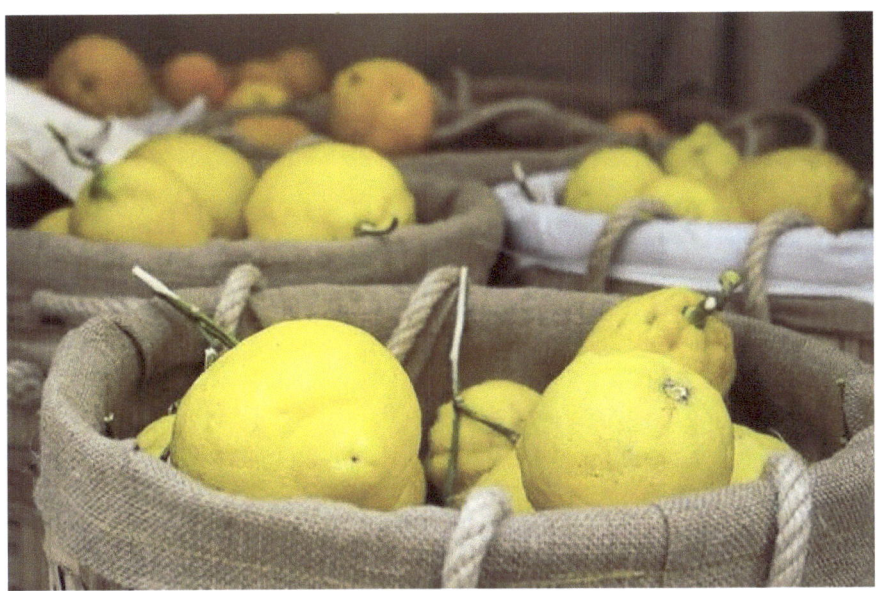

Chapter 7: Essential Oil Recipes

Peppermint and Lavender Swish

Make sure you buy ingestible lavender and peppermint. Take four ounces of water and drop two drops of lavender and two drops of lemon into the water. Swish it around in your mouth for about fifteen seconds and swallow. This recipe will help cure your allergies. Take daily during allergy season.

Lemon and Eucalyptus Steam

One of the best ways to beat allergies is with a lemon and eucalyptus steam. Put in one drop of eucalyptus and two drops of lemon essential oil in a half gallon water that has been boiled and poured into a bowl that can handle hot water. Then put a drop of each on a towel that will fit over your head and allow the steam to hit your face under the towel and the vapor from the essential oils will lovingly cure your allergies.

Lavender, Lemon, Eucalyptus, or Peppermint Rub

The easiest way to cure allergies is to rub essential oils on your chest, neck, and throat with the carrier oils jojoba or grape seed oil. You can mix one drop to an oz of carrier oil or more, enough to rub on all these areas. You can do it day and night for as long as allergy season lasts.

Lavender, Lemon, Eucalyptus, or Peppermint Shampoo

As well as rubbing the essential oils on the body, the hair is another place where the vapor action of eucalyptus, lavender, lemon, or peppermint can heal allergies for you. By buying a natural unscented shampoo or lotion and then adding about fifteen drops of just one or a combination of a few of these essential oils adding up to fifteen, will help heal your allergies.

Frankincense Amazing Massage Oil

Frankincense is an awesome smelling essential oil and a very effective essential oil with anti-inflammatory properties. Frankincense is effective on DNA. You can use frankincense for a wonderful massage oil to absorb through your skin and help you heal in many different ways. The recipe for this frankincense massage oil is one-half a cup of jojoba oil as you carrier oil and then eight drops of frankincense and four drops of lavender. This recipe creates wonderful smelling massage oil that you can put on yourself or use on someone else. You can buy empty lotion bottles at dollar stores or beauty care stores. You will mix your solutions in these bottles. Remember to label your bottles so you know exactly what is in them.

Bergamot, Rose, and Lime Room Spray

A beautiful room spray like bergamot, rose, and lime room spray is perfect to keep allergens down in your house. This wonderful room spray also makes you house smell fantastic after you have cleaned with one of the cleaning supply recipes down below. You can buy an eight ounce clean bottle from the beauty store that has a spray spout, and then put in about thirty-five drops of lime essential oil with about twenty-two drops of bergamot, and about four drops of rose. You will also need to add four ounces of distilled water to the bottle and mix around so that all the smells and wonderful oils blend to a beautiful mixture. Then simply spray in any one of your rooms and enjoy the lovely fragrance.

Rosemary and Grapefruit Room Spray

Another fantastic room spray is the recipe for rosemary and grapefruit. You simply use the water and bottle amount from above and then put in thirty-five Rosemary drops and fourteen grapefruit drops. Now you have a unique smelling room spray that is wonderful.

Lavender Carpet Fragrance

Carpets can so easily get dirty and stay that way. There are many harsh chemical carpet cleaners that you do not want to use when you are trying to cure allergies. A lovely carpet cleaner is to take a sixteen ounce of baking soda and twenty-five drops of lavender and put them together in a bowl. You want to mix it up well with a whisk or spoon. You may want to purchase a sifter that you use for flour in the kitchen or a very fine strainer and sift or lightly sprinkle the combination on your floor. You can leave on as long as you want. Then you will just vacuum as usual.

Lemon, Lavender, Clove, and Eucalyptus Counter Cleaner

The counters need to be cleaned, and you don't want to put chemicals on them, so this amazing recipe helps clean them up and leave them smelling fresh and beautiful. You simply take a cup of white vinegar and a cup of water and put in about six drops of each essential oil into a clean spray bottle and shake it up. You will then use the spray wherever there is a surface and let the solution stay on the surface a little bit, so the vinegar works into the dirt and bacteria that is on the surface. After about five to ten minutes, take your paper towel and wipe. What you have left behind is a beautiful clean smell void of chemicals.

Lavender or Lemon Bathroom Cleaner

The toilet is always a place where there are germs and the water in the toilet is a great way to scent up the place in a beautiful way. So with this great Lavender or Lemon recipe, you can allow the solution to sit in the toilet as long as you like to create a wonderful smell in the air. You will simply mix one cup of water and another cup of white vinegar and about twenty drops of either the lavender or the lemon and then put in the toilet bowl. You can use your brush to clean the toilet and then leave the solution in there for a while, so it cleans and freshens up the place.

Grapefruit Facial Toner

Beauty products are extremely expensive these days and don't always really smell that great. Making your facial toner will help alleviate allergies by using natural products and as well will help you save money and time. It also gives you something to do while you watch television or waiting for the casserole to be finished. You can buy a four ounce clean bottle from the beauty supply place and mix four ounces of hydrosol witch hazel with about sixteen drops of grapefruit essential oil plus eight drops of cypress essential oil, and then shake it up. Then you use a clean cotton ball and squeeze a small amount of toner on your cotton ball and wipe away your makeup as well as your dead skin after your facial cleansing.

As you can see, there are so many wonderful recipes to make when it comes to essential oils. The combinations are endless for what you can do with the essential oils. The best thing to do is to follow these recipes or go to the natural foods store closest to you, and they usually have testers so that you can smell each essential oil. You want to pick out your favorite ones and then use them in the recipes that you want. Between skin care, hair care, housing products, and internally, essential oils can be used in so many aspects of your life to help cure allergies. Remember to always use precaution as well. You can experiment yourself and come up with your own lovely combinations as well.

Essential oil recipes are fun and vast. These are just a few of the recipes that exist. Feel free to surf the web as well and find more great recipes. You can also mix your room freshener's with holiday scents like for Christmas and Easter while at the same time helping alleviate and cure allergies. Why not try a few recipes today.

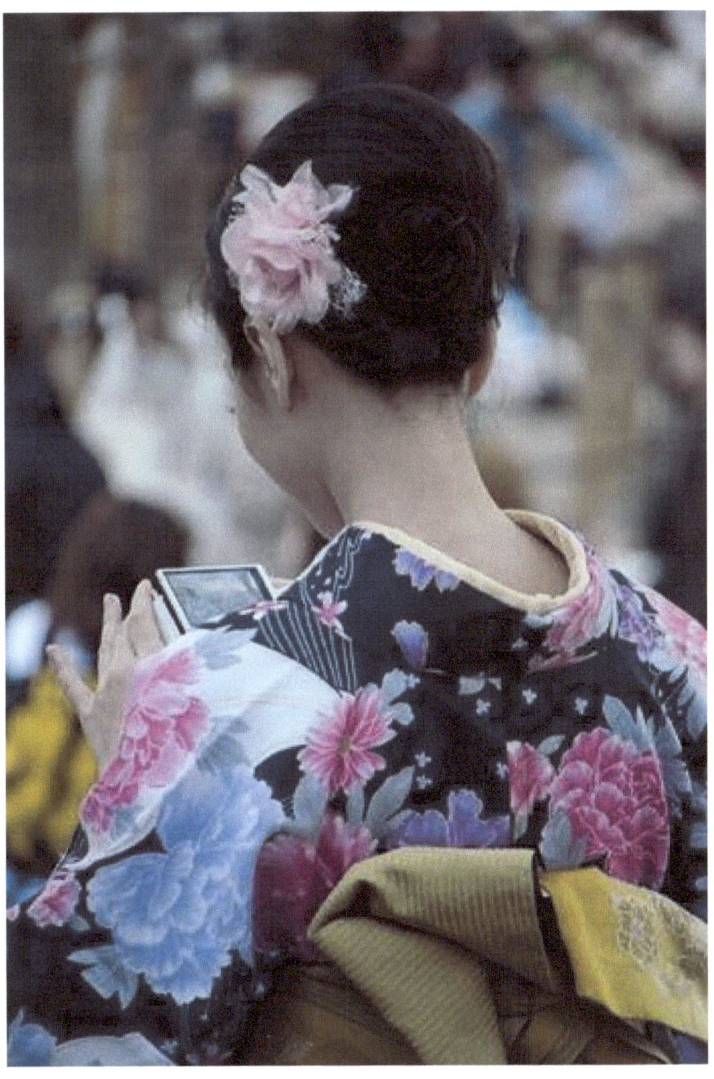

Grab Free Books Here

From time to time, I would highlight to my readers some interesting books which I found on Kindle. Subscribe to our newsletter to receive free bestselling kindle books recommendation delivered to your inbox daily. You can subscribe to our newsletter by clicking on the link below:

http://giveaway.kindleheaven.com/index.php/kindle-free-book/

It is 100% free and there will not be a single spam email. Just pure sharing of good books with my readers.

Please also like our facebook page below to get recommendation on good books to read for the day.

https://www.facebook.com/Kindle-Heaven-1651266215134798

Follow us on Twitter to get tweets on worthwhile books

https://twitter.com/KindleHeaven

Conclusion

Holistic health has been on the rise for many years now. Most of the healing solutions from holistic including essential oils have been working for years, yet with modern medicine people have gotten away from it. It is time to come back to holistic health. Essential oils can help cure allergies and help you live a long and happy life. The beautiful wonderful smell of essential oils is a bonus for using these wonderful natural combinations that happen to heal and keep your immune system running strong and well.

Sometimes the cure is in the source. It may seem odd that flowers and plants, the very thing that can cause allergies have the remedy to cure allergies. The high concentration of the flowers, fruits, and plant of eucalyptus, lavender, peppermint, and lemon are so effective in opening the breathing airways, that you will have wished you had known about essential oils sooner. Remember nature is not a one-time thing, where you can just rub these solutions once and you are done. No, it is necessary for you to take care of yourself for the rest of your life. Essential oils can help you take care of that.

It is of utmost importance that you take care of your insides as well as your outsides. Essential oils can help you with everything on the outside, and some essential oils can help you with the insides. It is very important for you to help the essential cure your allergies by doing some very important routines. These routines consist of you going to sleep at a regular time every night and getting at least six to eight hours a night. Six only if your body can handle that. You must also drink at least six glasses or eight ounces of water a day. Get the best water you can. The next important routine is to eat on a regular basis, at regular times, and about the same time every day.

The foods you put in your body are extremely important. You want to put the least amount of processed foods as well as the least amount of preservatives in your body. You want to put pure food like organic vegetables and fruit as well whole grain foods like rice, oatmeal, whole grain pasta, quinoa, and the like. When it comes to meats, the freshest and most organic you can find is really important. If you cannot buy organic because of price, just buy some non-organic. If you have to buy all conventional vegetables and fruits, that's fine as long as you are eating the fresh foods. It is of utmost importance for helping the essential oils and yourself cure allergies.

The combination of you using the wonderful essential oil recipes in this book and the quality by which you take care of yourself will help cure your allergies. You will be able to breathe easy and clear. Remember it takes a little effort from you and a little pampering of yourself. Feel wonderful and good about taking care of yourself and not suffering anymore. The universe wants you to be free and clear of ailments that keep you down. Essential oils are the perfect natural remedy to help you live long and breathe freely for the rest of your life.

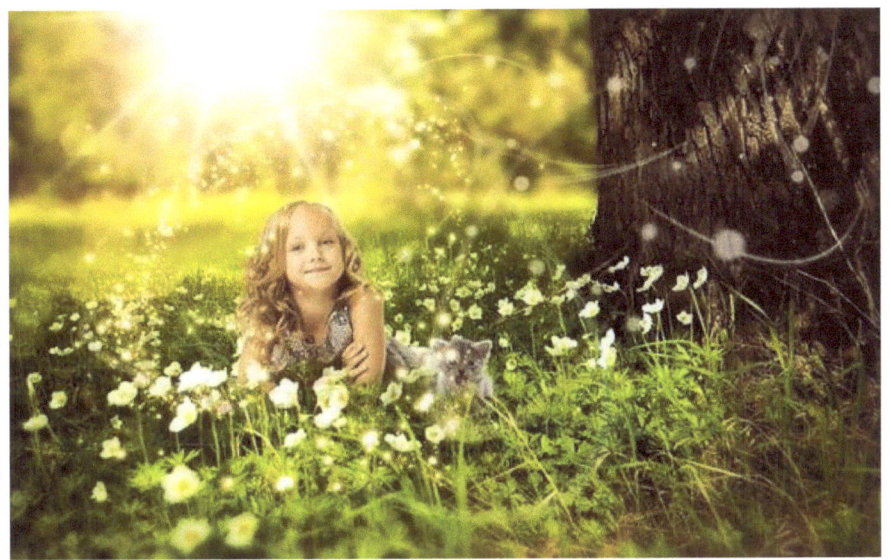

Thank you so much for reading this book, and I wish you the very best in life, allergy-free!

-   *Jeanne Hill*